The **Trustee** Guide to

BOARDROOM BASICS

in Health Care

James E. Orlikoff and Mary K. Totten

press

American Hospital Publishing, Inc.
An American Hospital Association Company
Chicago

This publication is designed to provide accurate and authoritative information in regard to the subject matter covered. It is sold with the understanding that neither the author nor the publisher is engaged in rendering legal, accounting, or other professional service. If legal advice or other expert assistance is required, the services of a competent professional should be sought.

The views expressed in this publication are strictly those of the authors and do not necessarily represent official positions of the American Hospital Association.

AHA is a service mark of the American Hospital Association used under license by American Hospital Publishing, Inc.

American Hospital Publishing, Inc., gratefully acknowledges the financial support of Witt/Kieffer · Ford · Hadelman · Lloyd for the initial development of these materials.

ISBN: 1-55648-221-3   Item Number: 196141

CONTENTS

ABOUT THE AUTHORS

James E. Orlikoff is president of Orlikoff & Associates, a Chicago-based consulting firm specializing in health care leadership, quality, and risk management. He was formerly the director of the American Hospital Association's Division of Hospital Governance and director of the Institute on Quality of Care and Patterns of Practice of the AHA's Hospital Research and Education Trust.

Mr. Orlikoff has been involved in quality, leadership, and risk management issues for over 10 years. He has designed and implemented hospital quality assurance and risk management programs in four countries and, since 1985, has worked with hospital governing boards to strengthen their overall effectiveness and their oversight of quality assurance and medical staff credentialing. He has written 6 books and over 40 articles and currently serves on hospital and civic boards.

Mary K. Totten is president of Totten & Associates, an Oak Park, Illinois–based consulting firm specializing in health care leadership. She was formerly program director for the Division of Hospital Governance of the American Hospital Association.

Ms. Totten has been a speaker and consultant to hospital and system boards, hospital associations, and managed care organizations on strategic planning and mission development, quality of care, medical staff credentialing, governance restructuring, and other governance issues. She has managed grant projects; published monographs, briefing papers, and articles for hospital trustees; and has worked with national trustee leaders to assess the governing board's responsibility for quality care. She has also developed discussion forums and publications on defining and measuring quality for health care purchasers and providers.

PREFACE

As consolidation continues in health care markets across the country, health care organization governing boards are taking time out to reexamine their structure and function to more effectively govern the evolving organizations they serve. As a result of such reevaluation, many boards are asking fundamental questions:

- What talents, skills, experience, and other attributes ought we to look for in the trustees we ask to serve on our governing boards?
- What are the basic roles and responsibilities of the board and of its individual members?
- Do we have a process in place to ensure that new board members, and our seasoned trustees, understand their governance responsibilities and the industry and organization in which they govern?

The Trustee *Guide to Boardroom Basics in Health Care* is a collection of three interactive chapters first published individually as workbooks in *Trustee* magazine. Together, "Board Composition and Trustee Selection," "Board Job Descriptions," and "Orientation: Basic Building Blocks of Effective Boards" begin at the beginning to help boards build a solid foundation for effective governance.

"Board Composition and Trustee Selection" addresses the issue of board size; discusses processes and criteria for selecting board members and reappointing existing members to the board; and explains board profiling—a technique boards can use to assess their current membership composition and strategically recruit new trustees.

"Board Job Descriptions" presents a rationale for developing board job descriptions; discusses the purposes job descriptions can fulfill; identifies a variety of governance roles and responsibilities that can be included in job descriptions; and presents examples of and suggestions for developing board, chairperson, and individual trustee job descriptions.

"Orientation: Basic Building Blocks of Effective Boards" looks at common characteristics of effective orientation processes; discusses why orientation is essential to good governance; and describes how to plan for and conduct meaningful orientation processes design to provide a strong foundation for ongoing trustee education and development.

The chapters begin with a topic overview, which is followed by discussion questions, exercises intended to help boards apply the material to their own situation, tips for improving governance effectiveness, and a self-assessment questionnaire to help boards diagnose their own strengths and weaknesses and identify areas for improvement.

The Trustee *Guide to Boardroom Basics in Health Care* can be used by the full board, board committees, or multidisciplinary leadership groups. Specific chapters can be used to explore a topic during time set aside for board education in conjunction with a regular board meeting or a board retreat. The board governance committee will find this book useful when planning and discharging its responsibilities for board member recruitment, and executives can use it to help plan for the implementation of specific recommendations for governance redesign that focus on the issues that this booklet covers. Finally, these workbooks can be used as part of a board self-evaluation to help assess and improve overall board performance.

While each chapter can be used interactively in a full-group setting, some exercises are designed to be completed by individual board members and then shared with the group as part of an educational or planning session. This approach helps orient board members to a specific topic in advance of group discussion and maximizes the time available for thoughtful interaction among group members.

We hope that *The* Trustee *Guide to Boardroom Basics in Health Care* becomes a staple among your governance resources and that it not only proves to be a key source of information for you but also a key that opens doors to learning from your fellow board members and leadership partners.

James E. Orlikoff and Mary K. Totten

1

Board Composition and Trustee Selection

Immediately after making a speech to a group of film students about his work, director John Huston was cornered by a critical student. "Mr. Huston, do you realize that at least 50 percent of the success of your films is simply due to good casting?" the student rudely asserted. Unflappable, Huston replied, "My boy, my films are *100 percent* good casting."

The moral of the story? John Huston was a great director partially because he realized that the cast he chose could make or break a film. The same can be said for a governing board: The members of the board, why and how they are chosen, and how their skills and backgrounds are balanced to complement one another will have a huge impact on the effectiveness of that board and the success of the organization it governs.

When hospitals were in a relatively stable environment, the demands upon and contributions required of a board were predictable. Boards were homogeneous and stable and rarely had limits on terms of office, so trustee selection was an infrequent activity.

But in today's environment, boards need to start considering many other factors, including

- size
- criteria for selecting and recruiting new members
- criteria for reappointing trustees to additional terms
- establishing terms and term limits
- establishing policies and procedures to address ongoing trustee recruitment and other board functions

■ establishing a board committee structure to perform these functions

Board Size

The proper size of a board depends on its roles and responsibilities. Nevertheless, the trend toward streamlining illustrates the emerging view that boards of fewer than 20 members tend to be more efficient.

Research suggests that the upper limit for effective and efficient group decision making is around 20 people. Anything larger can cause problems with communication and coordination, as well as the formation of factions and the diffusion of individual responsibility. The minimum size of a board depends on the number of members needed to provide a range of knowledge, skills, and experience.

Exercise: Board Size

Please read the following statements and answer the questions that follow. This exercise may be completed by individual trustees, then discussed with the entire board.

Following are arguments in favor of larger boards—those with more than 20 members:

■ increased ability to represent all segments of the community and the organization's constituencies
■ ability to spread the work among more members
■ ability to recruit affluent and politically connected people who will not participate in board functions other than raising funds and conducting political advocacy activities

Following are some arguments against larger boards:

■ more cumbersome decision making
■ less commitment and involvement on the part of board members
■ increased chance of "cliques" forming or power becoming vested in a subgroup of the board

Following are some arguments in favor of smaller boards—ones of 10 members or fewer:

- faster decision making
- more focus
- more flexibility
- fewer problems with communication and coordination

Following are some arguments against small boards:

- burnout as a result of trustees being spread too thin on board and committee work
- difficulty of achieving a good mix of skills, knowledge, and experience
- potential lack of depth if there is unexpected trustee turnover
- potential ability of one or two individuals to exert a disproportionate influence on the board's decisions

1. Which of the preceding arguments do and your board find more persuasive?
2. How large is your board? Is this size appropriate?
3. Why is your board this size?
4. Should the size of your board be modified? If so, how?

Who Should Be on the Board?

Obviously, the makeup of the board affects its function, so trustees should be chosen carefully. Further, the choice of members should be based on some type of criteria that takes into account the board's needs as well as the likely contributions of potential members.

But many boards do not have clearly articulated functions, so asking who should serve is putting the cart before the horse. Before trustees can be selected, the board as a whole needs to decide: What are we supposed to do? What individual skills, characteristics, and backgrounds of people will most effectively allow the board to do its job?

This progression is logical, but it's seldom simple. That's because most boards have many functions, some explicit, some implicit. Each function places different, and frequently contradictory, demands on board composition.

If a board is supposed to represent the community, for example, some would say that its membership should be a cross section of the community. If the board is supposed to exercise business acumen, that argues for trustees with business expertise. Trustees with backgrounds in health care may contribute to the board's function, but so might trustees with legal, accounting, or social service backgrounds, and so on.

Questions for Discussion

1. Why is your board composed as it currently is?
2. Why were you chosen to be a member?
3. Is the current makeup of the board ideal for addressing the changing issues, trends, and threats in health care?
4. As you survey the board, what skills are missing that will be needed to address the changing health care environment?
5. How many of your trustees are members of your organization's defined community? Is that number appropriate?
6. How is your governing board's composition different today than it was five years ago?
7. How will your board's composition likely be different five years from now?

Tips for Effective Governance Composition and Trustee Selection

- Clarify and articulate the board's functions and make them the foundation for the development of criteria for new trustee selection.
- Translate the functions of the board into a written job description that states roles and responsibilities.
- Develop a written trustee job description and use it as the basis for developing performance criteria to determine trustee reappointment.
- Establish a structured, integrated, and specific system of trustee selection, reappointment, and board composition.

- Develop a profile containing each board member's key characteristics, such as skills, experience, and background, in order to help identify gaps or areas of need on the board.
- Institute term limits for members of the board (for example, a three-year term with a maximum of three consecutive terms for a total of nine years of possible consecutive board membership).
- Systematically employ criteria for reappointment that assess all board members. Trustee terms should not be renewed automatically.
- Make the board a workable size—between 10 and 20 members.
- Assign responsibility to a board development or nominating committee to develop an integrated approach to trustee selection, reappointment, and board composition.
- Link the development of criteria for selecting new trustees to the annual board objectives, the work plan, and the organization's strategic plan.
- Annually evaluate the process, criteria, and priorities used to select and reappoint trustees and balance board composition.

Credentialing Trustees: A Future Trend?

As integrated delivery systems (IDSs) emerge, questions arise about the leadership skills, big-picture thinking, and political savvy necessary to effectively govern them. Some wonder if billion-dollar health systems should be governed by "amateur" trustees.

Doctors need credentialing before they can be appointed and reappointed to a medical staff, managed care panel, or physician-hospital organization (PHO). Will the trustees of tomorrow's IDSs and health care organizations need to be credentialed as well? Futurists like Russell C. Coile Jr. think so.

In the future, health systems may set very explicit criteria for system board membership. One such criterion could be past governance experience, according to evidence from a long-range study of nine IDSs.

This research study, conducted by Stephen Shortell, Ph.D., of Northwestern University, suggests that successful systems are governed by trustees who have already had experience at the hospital or other institutional board level.

Credentialing Criteria for Board Membership

Possible categories of criteria for member selection and reappointment include general qualifications criteria, demographic criteria, specific qualifications criteria, and position criteria.

Because all trustees must meet the general qualifications criteria, these should be applied fairly rigidly. For example, there is no point in selecting an otherwise wonderful trustee who cannot attend a majority of meetings, participate in group decision making, or keep confidential matters confidential.

Demographic criteria relate to such issues as the geographic location of board members, as well as the age, gender, and racial mix of the board. Typically, demographic criteria are used as flexible guidelines rather than rigid rules.

Specific qualifications criteria should reflect both the continuing and specific needs of a well-rounded board. It is in this category that knowledge, skills, experience, occupation, contacts, politics, affluence, and other characteristics are employed. Specific qualifications criteria are typically used to create a balance of skills, experience, and knowledge.

Finally, position criteria establish membership positions for individuals who hold specific jobs, usually within the organization. A typical example is a bylaws requirement that grants ex-officio membership (with voting power) to the hospital CEO and the chief of the medical staff.

Exercise: Trustee Selection Criteria

---

1. Please review the following sets of criteria, then rank those that would be most important when establishing an effective board for a health care organization of tomorrow. This may be done individually, then discussed with the entire board.
   - general qualifications criteria
     —willingness to serve on the hospital board
     —ability to meet the projected time commitment

—ability to function as a member of a deliberative body
—willingness to undergo board orientation and continuing education
—objectivity
—intelligence
—communication skills
—integrity and the absence of conflict of interest
—values

- demographic criteria
  —Should all trustees be required to live within certain geographical boundaries?
  —Should at least one trustee serve on the board who does not live in the organization's service area?
  —Should there be age parameters for membership (for example, a minimum age of 21 and a maximum of 75)?
  —Should an attempt be made to balance board membership on the basis of gender?
  —Should an attempt be made to balance board membership on the basis of race?

- specific qualifications criteria
  —prior experience on other boards (such as membership on the board of a hospital with at least 300 beds, a system with $50 million to $100 million in combined revenues, or a 50-plus physician medical group practice; or at least three years on the board of a large private-sector corporation or not-for-profit organization)
  —professional and business achievements
  —specific occupation and skills, such as business, medicine, law, or nursing
  —leadership skills
  —big-picture skills
  —systems thinking skills
  —a record of community involvement and commitment
  —political connections
  —experience in mergers in other organizations
  —experience in downsizing in other organizations
  —experience in reengineering in other organizations
  —experience as an executive or board member of a major health care purchaser (such as a large employer or local or county government)

- position criteria
  - —health care organization CEO
  - —other health care organization senior executives
  - —president of the PHO
  - —chair of the PHO board
  - —chair of the foundation
  - —chair of the auxiliary
2. Should criteria for reappointment to the board for additional terms be developed and used by the nominating or board development committee? Such criteria could include
   - minimum attendance requirements for board meetings
   - regular attendance at board committee meetings
   - meaningful participation at board and committee meetings
   - preparation in advance for meetings
   - attendance at a set minimum of board continuing education sessions
3. What other criteria or categories of criteria for board membership should be considered?

Board Profiling for Effective Composition and Trustee Selection

To get a picture of your board's profile, develop a chart that outlines the skills, qualifications, demographic characteristics, and tenure of each trustee. Use the chart or profile to identify gaps in the board—such as missing or redundant expertise or demographic characteristics.

You can then develop a profile of the characteristics and composition of an ideal board. Obviously, no one ideal board for all health care organizations exists. But the ideal can be compared with the profile of your current board, and differences between the two can form the basis for developing criteria for selecting and reappointing trustees.

Exercise: Board Profiling

1. Develop a profile of your board. For each member, list expertise, areas of interest, professional background, type and length of community involvement, age, residency, gender,

race, ethnicity, board tenure, and years remaining until the maximum term limit is reached. Now consider the following:

- What are the areas of duplication or member clustering on the board? (For example, it may be composed of a majority of white, 60-year-old bankers, with two years left until they reach the maximum term limit.)
- What are the demographic characteristics that are underrepresented on the board?
- Based on the board profile, what characteristics should be sought in the next three trustees you recruit?

2. Develop a profile of the "ideal" board for helping your organization achieve its strategic plan.
3. Compare your current board profile with your ideal. What differences exist between the two? Based upon these differences, what criteria for new trustee selection should your board develop and employ? What criteria for trustee reappointment should you develop or discard?

Board Composition and Trustee Selection: A Self-Assessment Questionnaire

The following survey addresses the board's responsibilities in selecting its own members and maintaining a proper trustee composition. It can be used as a stand-alone survey or as part of an overall board self-evaluation. Have each trustee independently and anonymously rate performance on the following questions. Compile and analyze all the responses and discuss them with the entire board. The discussion should result in an action plan to improve performance.

1. The current size of our board is appropriate and contributes to efficient and effective board performance.

   ❑ Strongly Agree ❑ Agree
   ❑ Somewhat Disagree ❑ Disagree

2. Bylaws determine our board's size.

   ❑ Strongly Agree ❑ Agree
   ❑ Somewhat Disagree ❑ Disagree

3. Board members are selected based on preestablished criteria.

   ❏ Strongly Agree   ❏ Agree
   ❏ Somewhat Disagree   ❏ Disagree

4. The board effectively identifies community leaders as potential new board members.

   ❏ Strongly Agree   ❏ Agree
   ❏ Somewhat Disagree   ❏ Disagree

5. We limit the tenure of our board members to focus commitment and gain new expertise.

   ❏ Strongly Agree   ❏ Agree
   ❏ Somewhat Disagree   ❏ Disagree

6. Reappointment depends on a review of the trustee's performance and is based on preestablished criteria.

   ❏ Strongly Agree   ❏ Agree
   ❏ Somewhat Disagree   ❏ Disagree

7. A particular committee oversees the process for selecting and reappointing trustees.

   ❏ Strongly Agree   ❏ Agree
   ❏ Somewhat Disagree   ❏ Disagree

8. When considering composition, we compare a profile of an ideal board with a profile of current members to identify needs, gaps, and redundancy.

   ❏ Strongly Agree   ❏ Agree
   ❏ Somewhat Disagree   ❏ Disagree

9. Our board is properly composed to lead us into the 21st century and to achieve our strategic plan.

   ❏ Strongly Agree   ❏ Agree
   ❏ Somewhat Disagree   ❏ Disagree

Conclusion

The members of the board, who they are, why they are chosen, whether they are reappointed to successive terms of office, all affect the function and effectiveness of the board and, ultimately, the organization.

As the health care environment changes, so does the character and function of governance. So, too, should the process of and criteria for selecting new board members.

2

Board Job Descriptions

There is one thing all boards have in common . . . they do not function.

—*Peter F. Drucker*

Tasks, Responsibilities, Practices

If we are unable to adequately describe what boards do, then how can we possibly hope to assess how well they do it?

—*Jeffrey A. Alexander, Ph.D., University of Michigan*

A health care governance consultant was asked recently, "If you could recommend only one thing to improve the performance of boards, what would it be?" Without hesitation he replied: "Job descriptions for boards, board members, and board leaders."

Why job descriptions? Because an extremely common cause of governance ineffectiveness is confusion among board members about what their roles and responsibilities are. Further, there is often confusion about the board's roles and responsibilities in relation to those of management, the medical staff, and other physician organizations; other boards; and committees of the board. Moreover, it is frequently unclear what the jobs of the board chair, committee chair, and board member are.

The most fundamental characteristic of excellent governance is that all board members have a shared understanding of their job. Every board has a somewhat different definition and allocation of its roles and responsibilities. Every board has a different mix of skills, personalities, and challenges. Every board must answer for itself the basic question: What is the job of the board of this health care organization?

The Purpose of Board Job Descriptions

Board job descriptions serve several important purposes, including

- *New board member recruitment:* Written board job descriptions help to focus the search for new trustees on individuals with the skills and talents that are most appropriate to the functions and needs of a board. More important, a well-written and up-to-date job description will let candidates know precisely what will be expected of them should they choose to join the board. Further, the job description tells potential candidates who have served on other boards the ways in which this one is unique.
- *New board member orientation:* A good position description details the role and work of the board and its members. This helps new members to become oriented more quickly and completely, to ask more informed questions, and to become more effective trustees.
- *Board self-evaluation:* Meaningful board self-evaluations are based upon a review of the effective discharge of the duties and responsibilities of the board. Thus, a board job description, along with annual board goals and objectives, provides a foundation for evaluating board performance.
- *Keeping governance on track:* A board job description allows board members to point out when a board is drifting away from performing some of its key roles and responsibilities. Further, it enables the board members to fine-tune the group's performance on an ongoing basis by comparing what the job description says the board should be doing with what it actually is doing.

- *Preventing conflict among multiple boards:* More than half of all U.S. health care organizations are part of corporate structures that have more than one board. Job descriptions help prevent conflict among multiple boards (for example, disputes about which board has the authority to do what) as well as decision-making gridlock (where decisions cannot be made without the approval of each board, creating inappropriately long decision-cycle times).
- *Clarifying the practical distinction between governance and management:* An effective board-CEO relationship, one that is framed by a mutual understanding of relative roles and responsibilities, is vital to the success of the health care organization. Unfortunately, this key relationship is often framed by implicit assumptions about relative roles, expectations, and job functions. A board job description (along with a CEO job description) helps both sides to understand and respect the limits of each other's responsibilities, as well as to identify areas of joint responsibility.

Questions for Discussion

1. If your board has a job description, which of the above purposes are achieved by it? Which are not? Why?
2. If your board doesn't have a job description, why not? What other mechanisms are used to clarify the board's roles and responsibilities? Are these mechanisms effective?

Governance Roles and Responsibilities

The terms *roles* and *responsibilities* are often used interchangeably when describing the job of a board; there is, however, a difference. *Responsibilities* refers to what a board does or should do; *roles* refers to how the board does it. A meaningful job description should first outline the primary responsibilities of the board and then review the roles of the board in discharging those responsibilities. While roles, or how a board accomplishes its duties, will vary, the first step in creating a meaningful job description is to achieve agreement on the board's most important responsibilities.

Exercise: Potential Board Responsibilities

Consider the following potential board responsibilities, then answer the questions that follow. The board

- defines and pursues the mission and safeguard the values of the organization
- selects, monitors, supports, evaluates, and compensates the CEO
- establishes long-term direction through oversight of and participation in strategic planning
- promotes financial viability via budget and financial oversight, fund development, and investment management
- maintains and continuously improves the quality of care and services of the organization
- monitors the effectiveness of significant organizational programs and takes action where appropriate to improve, modify, or eliminate such programs as necessary to maintain organizational excellence
- oversees and promotes positive relationships with the medical staff and physician organizations
- promotes and maintains positive external relationships with the community, local business, government, funding sources, and other health-related organizations
- assures that the health care organization meets regulatory, accreditation, and legal requirements
- oversees effective governance, including trustee recruitment, selection, and orientation; board education and self-evaluation; and effective function and structure
- acts with the highest integrity to advance the best interests of the organization and achieve its mission
- represents the community
- oversees philanthropic fund-raising and participates in fund development through contributions
- sets policies for the organization
- serves as adviser to the CEO
- is an advocate for and provides links to specific constituent groups
- appoints and reappoints physicians to the medical staff and delineates their privileges
- represents the interests of the sponsoring religious order or owner

Questions for Discussion

1. Of these governance responsibilities, which are most important? Why?
2. Are there any governance responsibilities that are not mentioned above that you believe are important? Identify them and add them to the list.
3. If you were to choose only five of the above responsibilities to form the basis of a job description for your board, which would you pick? Why?
4. Make sure that all the members of your board, or the members of the committee charged with drafting a job description for your board, answer question 3. Did they all choose the same responsibilities? If yes, you have the basis of the job description for your board. If not, which were chosen most often? This should form the basis of a board discussion as you develop a board job description.
5. What role should the board play in discharging each of its responsibilities? For example, should the board initiate, lead, or respond to a given situation? Will the board discharge its quality oversight responsibility as a committee of the whole or use a committee to review such issues as physician credentialing or the use of quality indicators and make recommendations to the full governing board?

Exercise: Board Job Description

Below are three summaries of actual board job descriptions. Review them and then answer the questions that follow.

Memorial Hospital Board Job Description

Primary objective: The board is responsible for the success of the organization—both the quality of care and financial viability.
  Governance responsibilities:

- adopt the mission and determine the scope of services to be offered
- approve long-range plans
- select, support, and advise the CEO

- establish and maintain procedures for effective governance, including board member selection, orientation, education, and self-evaluation
- assure that quality care is provided and oversee the medical staff credentialing process
- serve as an advocate for the hospital in the community

General Hospital Board Job Description

The board's primary responsibility is to develop and follow the mission. This involves development and oversight of policy in four vital areas:

1. quality and performance improvement
2. financial performance
3. effective planning
4. effective management performance

To accomplish these responsibilities, the board

- establishes policy guidelines for mission implementation and achievement, as well as mission evaluation
- evaluates proposals to ensure that they are consistent with the mission
- monitors existing programs and activities of the hospital to ensure that they are consistent with the mission
- periodically reviews and, if necessary, revises the mission to ensure that it is relevant to the changing environment

Community Hospital Board Job Description

The board provides governance oversight for programmatic and policy-related aspects of all hospital services and corporate activities consistent with the Articles of Incorporation. The board also appoints the CEO and approves all actions that the executive committee takes in the name of the board between meetings.

Further, the board adopts and adheres to statements of mission, vision, strategy, and values that are reviewed on a regular basis. It considers the health requirements of the community and how the hospital can meet them. The board determines the scope of programs and services and the desired levels of quality and provides advice and counsel to the CEO in the implementation of plans and programs.

Questions for Discussion

1. Of the three summary job descriptions, which did you think was the best? Which did you think was the worst? Why?
2. Which description would provide the best guidance to a board that is struggling to focus its activities?
3. Are there components of all three job descriptions that have value? If so, what are they and why?

Board Chair Job Descriptions

For the same reasons that a written job description can help improve the board's performance, a job description for the board chairperson can help improve the leadership and overall effectiveness of the board. In fact, much of a board's effectiveness and development will depend upon the quality of its leadership. Unfortunately, one of the problems with many board leadership positions is a total lack of definition of what the chair is supposed to do. When this is the case, the effectiveness of the board often varies as board chairs change. Personality, rather than principle, dictates board function and focus.

Another common problem with the job of board chairperson is little or no formal orientation to or training for the job. That, of course, is directly related to the absence of a job description, which would form the basis for the orientation.

A significant benefit of a chair job description is that it enables the board to hold the person accountable for specific responsibilities and actions. The "it's not my job" defense, frequently used in delicate situations such as disciplining an errant board member, cannot be employed in the face of a job description that clearly defines the responsibility or action as part of the job. As with the board, the first step in constructing a job description for the chairperson is to delineate the responsibilities.

Exercise: Chairperson Responsibilities

Consider the following potential responsibilities of a board chair, then answer the questions that follow. The board chair

- keeps the mission of the organization foremost and articulates it as the basis for all board action
- understands and communicates the role and functions of the board, committees, medical staff, and management
- understands and communicates individual board member, board leader, and committee chair responsibilities and accountability
- acts as liaison between the board, management, and the medical staff
- plans agendas and meetings of the general board and executive committees
- presides over the meetings of the board and executive committee
- presides over or attends other board, medical staff, and other organization meetings
- enforces board and hospital bylaws, rules, and regulations (such as conflict-of-interest and confidentiality policies)
- appoints board committee chairs and members consistent with a systematic approach
- acts as a liaison between and among other boards in the health care system
- establishes board goals and objectives and translates them into annual work plans
- directs the committees of the board, ensuring that the committee works plans flow from and support the hospital and board goals, objectives, and work plans
- orientates new board members and arranges continuing education for the board
- ensures that effective board self-evaluation occurs
- builds cohesion among the leadership team of the board chair, CEO, and medical staff leader
- leads the CEO performance objective and evaluation process
- plans for board leadership succession

1. Of these board chairperson responsibilities, which do you think are most important? Why?

2. Are there any responsibilities that are not mentioned above that you believe are important? Identify them and add them to the list.
3. If you were to choose only five of the above responsibilities to form the basis of a job description for your board chairperson, which would you pick? Why?
4. Make sure that all the members of your board, or the members of the committee charged with drafting a job description for your board chair, answer question 3. Did they all choose the same five responsibilities? If yes, you have the basis of the board chairperson job description. If not, which responsibilities were chosen most frequently? This should form the basis of a board discussion as you develop a chairperson job description.

Trustee Job Descriptions

While some health care organizations have a job description for the board and perhaps even the chairperson, few have a job description for the individual board members. This is a major contributor to ineffective governance because many boards are composed of members who have very different ideas about what being a trustee means. In essence, these trustees each have implicit and wildly divergent job descriptions in their heads that cause them to act differently from one another and to regard the behavior of their colleagues as inappropriate.

Exercise: Developing Trustee Job Descriptions

Develop a list of possible trustee responsibilities. These might include

- attending all board and committee meetings
- reviewing all agenda materials in advance of the meetings
- completing new board member orientation
- keeping board deliberations confidential
- abiding by the vote of the majority
- communicating with the media and constituent groups

Once developed, rank the responsibilities from most important to least important. Have each trustee do this and compare the individual responses. From the comparison, develop a master list and ranking of individual board member responsibilities. This will then serve as both the foundation and bulk of the trustee job description.

Tips on Developing and Using Meaningful Board Job Descriptions

- Identify and prioritize the responsibilities and roles of the board. Translate these into a written job description of no more than three pages in length.
- Make certain that the board job description covers every aspect of the board's responsibilities and functions.
- Develop job descriptions for the chair and the individual member positions.
- Use the written job descriptions for the individual board member as the basis for developing performance criteria to determine reappointment to additional terms on the board.
- Use the chairperson job description to develop selection criteria and evaluate performance.
- Place the board job description, along with those of the chair and trustee, in each board agenda book.
- Routinely compare how the board is functioning with how the job description says it should function and note and discuss significant differences between the description and actual performance.
- Use the job description as a foundation for new trustee orientation and new board leadership training programs.
- As part of annual board self-evaluation, assess the appropriateness and value of the job descriptions. Refine or revise the job description as appropriate.

A Self-Assessment Questionnaire

The following brief survey can be used as a stand-alone survey or as part of an overall board self-evaluation process. Each board member should independently and anonymously rate the board's performance on the issues detailed in the following questions. The responses should be compiled, analyzed, and then discussed with the entire board present. The board should pay particular attention to those questions with significant variation in responses and those with predominately negative responses.

1. Does the board have a written job description for itself?

   ❏ Yes   ❏ No

   For individual board members?   ❏ Yes   ❏ No

   For the board chairperson?   ❏ Yes   ❏ No

2. The relative responsibilities, roles, and authority of the multiple boards in our corporate structure or health care system are spelled out in job descriptions for each board.

   ❏ Strongly Agree   ❏ Agree
   ❏ Somewhat Disagree   ❏ Disagree

3. The roles and responsibilities of our board are clearly defined in relation to those of the other boards within our health care system or organization.

   ❏ Strongly Agree   ❏ Agree
   ❏ Somewhat Disagree   ❏ Disagree

4. The board and CEO agree on their relative roles and responsibilities, and these are reflected in job descriptions for the board and CEO.

   ❏ Strongly Agree   ❏ Agree
   ❏ Somewhat Disagree   ❏ Disagree

5. Board and trustee job descriptions are shared with potential new board members as part of the trustee recruitment process.

   ❏ Strongly Agree   ❏ Agree
   ❏ Somewhat Disagree   ❏ Disagree

6. Board and trustee job descriptions are the basis for new board member orientation.

   ❏ Strongly Agree   ❏ Agree
   ❏ Somewhat Disagree   ❏ Disagree

7. Board job descriptions are reviewed as part of board leader training and development activities.

   ❏ Strongly Agree   ❏ Agree
   ❏ Somewhat Disagree   ❏ Disagree

8. Responsibilities of our board and individual members, as outlined in their job descriptions, are assessed as part of our board's ongoing self-evaluation process.

   ❏ Strongly Agree   ❏ Agree
   ❏ Somewhat Disagree   ❏ Disagree

9. The board annually reviews and revises its job description.

   ❏ Strongly Agree   ❏ Agree
   ❏ Somewhat Disagree   ❏ Disagree

Conclusion

Written job descriptions focus a board's efforts on performing the governance functions of a health care organization, as opposed to its managerial functions. Job descriptions for the board as a whole, for the chairperson, and for the individual board members clarify the rights and responsibilities of each and, in the ideal, resolve conflicts before they arise.

3

Orientation: Basic Building Blocks of Effective Boards

In the past, people invited to join a health care organization board would often protest that they knew nothing about health care or what a hospital or system board does. "Just come to the meetings and you'll pick it up pretty quickly," they were frequently told. Unfortunately, this "learn as you go," or "osmosis" approach to trustee orientation is still common today and, paradoxically, usually results in years of trustee disorientation. So this method is actually counterproductive to effective governance.

When hospitals were in a relatively unchallenged environment, characterized by predictability and stability, the contributions of, and the need for, a board were questionable. Boards did not contribute much (other than philanthropic giving) to the governance of their facilities. If effective boards were not necessary to hospitals, effective trustees were certainly not necessary to hospital boards. So there was little, if any, need for meaningful trustee orientation.

Now hospitals and other health care organizations exist in a challenging, changing, and turbulent environment, so it has become clearer that the board and the way it functions influences the viability of the hospital it governs. More specifically the board can affect the hospital in one of two broad ways: It can either be an asset or it can be a liability.

One characteristic of an effective board is the existence of a meaningful trustee orientation process that all new board members go through. Orientation should depend on more than luck, exhortations to read thick and boring manuals, individual initiative, and "osmosis." It should be a planned, deliberate process based partly on the board's stated functions, goals, and objectives and partly on the culture, values, and history of the entity.

Introduction to New Trustee Orientation

What is an effective orientation? It's more than simply a mechanism for providing new trustees with information. It's a structured process for beginning the complete development of the board member. While there is no specific orientation method that will work for all boards, effective orientation processes share a number of characteristics:

- understanding of the overall purpose of orientation
- clear distinction of the relative roles and responsibilities for orientation (in other words, who does what)
- clearly defined curriculum for the orientation process that directly relates to the hospital and board
- clearly defined mechanism and time frame for conducting the orientation
- ongoing evaluation of the orientation process that results in regular refinements and occasional revisions

What Is the Purpose of the Orientation Process?

If the purpose of the orientation process is not clear, it probably won't achieve much. Asking the purpose is likely to spark an obvious answer: to orient the new board member, of course. But orient the new trustee to what? Because many trustee orientations are not based on an answer to this explicit question, most are remarkably ineffective.

While each health care organization will determine its own purpose for trustee orientation, several broad purposes are common, including

- providing a general overview of the health care field to give new trustees a context in which the organization exists and functions

- outlining the culture, values, and norms of the organization and showing how the board recognizes and acts to perpetuate these key organizational characteristics
- providing a sense of the hospital's or system's history to help new trustees contribute to continuity in governance
- grounding new trustees in the organization's strategy as well as familiarizing them with the specific market characteristics that led to the development of the current strategic plan
- preparing new trustees for future board decisions and issues by reviewing local market trends
- providing new trustees with a solid picture of the hospital's finances
- reviewing recent, significant board decisions and their impact
- reviewing the structure, function, bylaws, and policies and procedures of the board, as well as its roles and responsibilities and those of any other boards within the organization
- providing an understanding of board values and culture and how they specifically affect the governance process
- reviewing the relationship of the organization to physicians and physician organizations as well as to other key constituency groups

Questions for Discussion

1. Which of the preceding purposes of orientation programs are the most important? Why?
2. Which of the purposes were achieved or addressed in your organization's trustee orientation process? Which were not?
3. How should your orientation process be modified to address any additional purposes you have identified?

Conducting Trustee Orientation

After the purposes of a new trustee orientation process are established, the next step is to determine who will conduct and oversee the process. This job often falls solely on the shoulders of the CEO. While it is appropriate for the CEO to be heavily involved in, and perhaps lead, the orientation process, remember that trustee orientation is a key component of board development. That's why the board should oversee the orientation process through a committee like the executive or board development committee.

A crucial component of the process is making newcomers feel comfortable with the board and the way it functions. Board members should also be involved in conducting key aspects of the process itself. Involvement of the board chair and several experienced trustees, as well as the chair of the committee to which the new trustee is likely to belong, is therefore desirable.

It is also appropriate to have outgoing trustees meet with newcomers to contribute a sense of continuity, or "passing the baton." In fact, by structuring the orientation process in order to coincide or conclude with a board retreat or board development session, the board as a whole can contribute to the orientation of new trustees.

One productive technique is for new trustees to attend a board self-evaluation session as soon as possible after they join the board. By participating in such a session, new trustees can see how the board examines and structures its function and how it evaluates its strengths and weaknesses. They'll also learn about board values and internal relationships among trustees and between the board and the CEO.

New trustees will be able to interact with other trustees outside the structure of board meetings, thereby building relationships, rapport, and board cohesiveness. Participation in a board self-evaluation session or retreat is an excellent way to accomplish what could otherwise take a year or more.

Besides retreats, other mechanisms for trustee orientation can include lectures, meetings, videotapes, written material, one-on-one discussions, tours of physical facilities, "auditing" various board committee meetings, and attendance at outside education programs.

One technique that many boards find particularly effective is pairing each new trustee with a seasoned trustee mentor. This approach not only gives new trustees specific resources for questions over time, but it can help provide a role model for new board members to observe effective governance in action. Furthermore, it signals to other trustees on the board that the mentors are those who have successfully mastered the techniques of good governance.

Questions for Discussion

1. Who conducts the trustee orientation in your facility? Why?
2. Who else could be involved in your orientation process to make it better?
3. Is the process overseen by the board as a whole or by a board committee, such as the board development, governance, or executive committee?
4. How long does a new trustee sit on your board before a retreat is held? Is this time frame appropriate?

Orientation Content

The next component of an effective trustee orientation process is a clearly defined curriculum. A meaningful orientation curriculum should be directly related to the mission and strategic direction of the health care organization and to board function and structure. But first the orientation process should provide a broad understanding of the health care field.

A number of issues should be reviewed to form this broad base:

- U.S. health care: its history, financing, and delivery and the reasons for, and impact of, the massive changes in the system; a review of payers and payment mechanisms, emphasizing the transition from fee-for-service to managed care and capitation
- hospitals and integrated delivery systems in general and within the context of the health care field
- the history and evolution of hospital and health care governance, including the legal authority and responsibilities of the board and its members and regulatory requirements
- physicians in the context of changes in health care, including the stress and pressures on doctors: loss of autonomy, reduced income, and increased scrutiny; the formation of

physician groups; and the relationship of physician groups to hospitals and purchasers
- the evolution of, and changes in, the medical staff, including its roles and responsibilities, and the changing relationship of the physician to the medical staff and of the medical staff to the hospital and board
- current health care trends and predicted future directions

Once this general orientation has been completed, conduct an orientation to the specifics of the organization and its governance. This orientation should review and discuss

- the history, mission, and values of the organization
- organizational structure, including a succinct review of hospital and medical staff bylaws
- hospital and system programs and services
- specific roles and responsibilities of the board, including a review of board policies and structure
- specific types of information (such as financial and quality reports) that will be routinely reported to the board and how to interpret this information
- hospital management roles, responsibilities, and structure
- medical staff roles, responsibilities, and structure
- the strategic plan and its current implementation status
- analysis of critical board relationships: boards of related corporations, subsidiaries, or parent
- review of board liability issues and protections

Once the orientation content is developed, determine the mechanisms and time frame for conducting the actual orientation: lectures, meetings, videotapes, written materials, retreats, one-on-one discussions, tours of physical facilities, "auditing" various board committee meetings, pairing each new trustee with a seasoned trustee mentor, and attendance at outside education programs.

In general, the more mechanisms used, the more effective the overall orientation process will be. Don't simply give new trustees a thick orientation manual and instruct them to "feel free to ask questions."

A meaningful orientation should not be a one-time event. Instead it should be constructed as an ongoing process over a period of several months, using various mechanisms and formats. But the process should not mark completion of the board's or new members' education. Ongoing education is a cornerstone of board development and effective governance, especially in today's turbulent climate. Activities that often are part of ongoing board education and development programs include

- attending regular leadership retreats
- devoting part of each board meeting to education on a specific topic
- sending board members to external educational programs
- subscribing to publications
- using audio- or videotapes designed for health care organization board members
- conducting periodic board self-assessments

Furthermore, just as the changing environment requires constant adjustment in the planning, structure, and operation of the health organization, it also requires continual change in the organization and operation of the governing board.

That's why the new trustee orientation process should be evaluated to make sure it is effective in preparing trustees for their demanding roles and modified as various changes in the health care field, the hospital, and the process of governance occur.

Questions for Discussion

1. Which of the broad health care issues and organization-specific information mentioned above are included in your orientation process?
2. What other issues are included? Should other issues be included?
3. How many of the learning formats and mechanisms mentioned in the previous section does your orientation program include? Which approaches do your board members find most effective?
4. When was your board's orientation process last evaluated or changed?

Tips for Effective Orientation Programs

- Make a point of involving board members in the new trustee orientation process.
- Charge a board committee to design, oversee, and periodically reevaluate the trustee orientation process.
- Ensure that the orientation process fulfills specific purposes or objectives and that these are regularly reviewed, modified as appropriate, and used to evaluate the overall effectiveness of the process.
- Ask new trustees to evaluate the orientation process after completing it. Also, ask trustees who have at least one to three years' experience on the board to think back to their own orientation process and suggest any additional topics that might have been helpful to new members. Then use this feedback in the overall trustee-orientation evaluation process.
- Schedule the trustee recruitment and orientation process to coincide with the annual board retreat so that a new board member can attend the retreat within the first three months of becoming a board member.
- Ensure that the orientation process offers pertinent information on the health care field in general and specific information on your health organization and its governance. In addition, ensure that the orientation process exposes new trustees to other board members and to leaders within the organization in ways that allow for socializing and building relationships.
- Use as many different mechanisms and formats as possible to convey information during the process.
- Support new trustee orientation with an ongoing program of board education and development.

A Self-Assessment Questionnaire

This brief survey addresses the board's roles and responsibilities in overseeing the orientation process. It can be used as a stand-alone survey or as part of an overall board self-evaluation.

Each trustee should independently and anonymously rate the board's performance on each of the following questions. Compile and analyze all the responses of the board and then discuss them with the entire board. Pay particular attention to questions that have significant variation in responses (where some trustees rate board performance high and some rate it low) and those questions with predominately negative responses.

1. Does the board have a formal new trustee orientation process?

   ❏ Yes   ❏ No

2. Are all new board members required to complete the process?

   ❏ Yes   ❏ No

3. Our new orientation process fulfills a specific purpose(s) or objective(s).

   ❏ Strongly Agree   ❏ Agree
   ❏ Disagree   ❏ Strongly Disagree

4. Our trustee orientation process provides information on broad health care issues and trends as well as information that is specific to our health care organization and its governance structure and function.

   ❏ Strongly Agree   ❏ Agree
   ❏ Disagree   ❏ Strongly Disagree

5. Several board members are involved in planning and conducting our process.

   ❏ Strongly Agree   ❏ Agree
   ❏ Disagree   ❏ Strongly Disagree

6. Our board orientation process includes opportunities to meet and socialize with other board members and organizational leaders.

   ❏ Strongly Agree   ❏ Agree
   ❏ Disagree   ❏ Strongly Disagree

7. The board, either as a whole or through one of its committees, is responsible for the design, conduct, and oversight of the process.

   ❏ Strongly Agree   ❏ Agree
   ❏ Disagree   ❏ Strongly Disagree

8. The board periodically evaluates the content, format, and process of board member orientation against the objectives it was designed to fulfill to ensure it continues to effectively meet its purpose(s).

❑ Strongly Agree   ❑ Agree
❑ Disagree   ❑ Strongly Disagree

9. The process is complemented and reinforced by board retreats and by an ongoing program of education and development.

❑ Strongly Agree   ❑ Agree
❑ Disagree   ❑ Strongly Disagree

10. Our current orientation process helps prepare new trustees to effectively lead our health care organization into the 21st century and to achieve our strategic goals.

❑ Strongly Agree   ❑ Agree
❑ Disagree   ❑ Strongly Disagree

11. The orientation process includes a component on the responsibility of the organization to its community and to the assessment and improvement of community health.

❑ Strongly Agree   ❑ Agree
❑ Disagree   ❑ Strongly Disagree

Conclusion

A meaningful new board member orientation process is a critical characteristic of effective governance. Just as a board will either help or hurt the organization it governs, so does a trustee either help or hurt the board to which he or she belongs. Successful boards and CEOs recognize this by constructing and conducting a formal and complete new trustee orientation process to get them off to the right start. They also regularly evaluate the process.

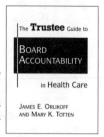
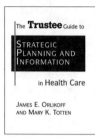
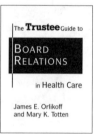
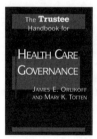